Thomas Dimsdale

Thoughts on General and Partial Inoculations

Containing a translation of two treatises written when the author was at

Petersburg, and published there in the Russian language; also outlines of

two plans.

Thomas Dimsdale

Thoughts on General and Partial Inoculations
*Containing a translation of two treatises written when the author was at
Petersburg, and published there in the Russian language; also outlines of two plans.*

ISBN/EAN: 9783337298272

Printed in Europe, USA, Canada, Australia, Japan

Cover: Foto ©ninafisch / pixelio.de

More available books at **www.hansebooks.com**

THOUGHTS

ON

GENERAL AND PARTIAL

INOCULATIONS.

CONTAINING

A Translation of Two Treatises written when the Author was at Petersburg, and published there, by Command of her Imperial Majesty, in the Russian Language.

ALSO

OUTLINES OF TWO PLANS:

One, for the general Inoculation of the Poor in small Towns and Villages.

The other, for the general Inoculation of the Poor in London, and other large and populous Places.

BY THE HONOURABLE

Baron THOMAS DIMSDALE,

First Physician and Actual Counsellor of State to her Imperial Majesty the Empress of all the Russias, and F. R. S.

LONDON:

Printed by WILLIAM RICHARDSON;

For W. OWEN, in Fleet-street; and T. CARNAN and F. NEW-bery jun. Nº 65, in St. Paul's Church-yard.

M.DCC.LXXVI.

[Price One Shilling and Six Pence.]

TO THE

LEGISLATURE

OF

GREAT BRITAIN,

THESE TRACTS,

ON A SUBJECT EXTREMELY INTERESTING
TO THE COMMUNITY,

ARE MOST RESPECTFULLY ADDRESSED BY

THE AUTHOR.

INTRODUCTION.

TO preserve the lives and health of the inferior part of mankind has been an object carefully attended to in all civilized and well regulated ftates, not only from motives of compaffion, but becaufe it has been plainly demonftrated that it is the intereft of the wealthy in every nation to encourage population, and provide for the wants of the poor.

One would indeed, on the firft thought prefume, that the unavoidable neceffities of the indigent would be voluntarily relieved out of the abundance of their opulent neighbours; but the number of laws that

a   have

have been made for the provifion of
the poor, are proofs of the futility
of this expectation, and the neceffity of compulfion.

Among the many objects that
have been provided for, it feems
matter of aftonifhment that no one
hás ever pointed out the Small Pox
as a diftemper, whofe deftructive
confequences might be in great mea-
fure prevented by the interpofition of
Legiflature, and the affiftance that
would be certainly afforded from
private charity.

It is now above fifty years fince
Inoculation was introduced into this
country, and like other new infti-
tutions was then oppofed; but at
prefent, though it may be impoffible
to define the numbers that are yearly
inoculated, it is certain that moft of
the wealthy approve and avail themfelves

felves of the practice: yet we view the Bills of Mortality with uncon- cern, though they demonftrate that the number of deaths from this dif- eafe is confiderably increafed; and with the affecting circumftance, that they are probably of the younger part of the people.

Although this matter has not been attended to here, it did not efcape the penetration of the Emprefs of Ruffia; who, with a regard to the happinefs of her people that deferves much greater commendation than I am able to beftow, was extremely folicitous to render Inoculation ge- neral among her fubjects: and it was with a view to this that foon after the recovery of the Emprefs and Grand Duke from this operation, her Majefty was pleafed to command me to write their cafes, with the principal occurrences during the Ino-

culation,

culation, from an idea that being publiſhed they would tend to the removal of prejudices, and the advancement of a practice ſhe had much at heart to encourage.

Her Imperial Majeſty alſo frequently did me the honor to converſe freely on ſeveral points reſpecting the natural Small Pox and Inoculation; and having been pleaſed to approve of the manner in which her enquiries and doubts were anſwered, I was afterwards commanded at different times to give in writing the ſubſtance of what had been advanced on theſe occaſions. Theſe orders were obeyed, the tracts tranſlated into the Ruſſian language, and as I imagined, were only intended for the peruſal of the Empreſs. But in the year 1770, my treatiſe on Inoculation, with the following tracts,

was

was publifhed at Peterfburg by her Majefty's command:

I. An Account of the Inoculation for the Small Pox of her Imperial Majefty, Autocratrix of all the Ruffias.

II. An Account of the Inoculation for the Small Pox of his Imperial Highnefs the Grand Duke, the Heir of all the Ruffias, by Baron Thomas Dimfdale, firft Phyfician to her Imperial Majefty.

III. Remarks on the Book, intitled, The prefent Method of Inoculating for the Small Pox, written by the Author now at St. Peterfburg.

IV. A fhort Defcription of the Methods propofed for extending the falutary Practice of Inoculation through

through the whole Ruffian Empire.

V. **A** fhort Eftimate of the Numbers of thofe who die of the natural Small Pox, with a View to demonftrate the Advantages that may accrue to Ruffia from the Practice of Inoculation, &c.

A tranflation of thefe tracts, with fome further remarks on Inoculation, and a relation of my journey to Ruffia, has been preparing for the Prefs; but on fome accounts unneceffary to be entered on here, is deferred.

Indeed, my appearance as a writer now is earlier than I intended, on account of a plan that I have feen of a Difpenfary for inoculating the poor of London at their own houfes, in which fome plaufible reafons for

fuch

fuch an eftablifhment are advanced; but I think they are much more fpecious than fubftantial; and that the plan itfelf is fraught with very dangerous confequences to the community, and not like to anfwer any good purpofe if put in execution. Wherefore I thought it a duty owing to the public to publifh thefe fentiments on the fubject, that none fhould inadvertently mifapply their charity fo as to do mifchief when good was intended.

In purfuance of this defign, it feemed not improper to begin with the two laft of the tracts that were wrote at Peterfburg in the year 1768, as my opinions on the fubjects treated of remain the fame as at that time. But I defire that what is advanced in them, or may be found in the fequel, that tends to difcountenance the practice of Inoculation by perfons who

who have not had a medical education, may not be conſtrued as a deſign to affect any of the family to
whoſe mode of practice Inoculation
is indebted for ſome conſiderable
improvements; nothing can be farther from my intention, for I have
been at all times diſpoſed to do them
juſtice, and allow all the merit that
is their due.

In fact, I am an advocate for
Inoculation; and wiſh the deſign of
extending the benefit to the poor
may be ſo conducted, as to afford
its enemies as few opportunities of
objecting to it on any ſolid ground
as poſſible; and that the affair may
be ſo well underſtood, as to make it
plain in what manner charitably diſpoſed perſons may moſt uſefully employ their benevolence.

A Description of the

METHODS

PROPOSED

For extending the falutary practice
of Inoculation through the whole
Ruffian Empire.

*Written at Peterfburg by her Imperial Ma-
jefty's firft Phyfician Baron* THOMAS
DIMSDALE.

In Obedience

AGREEABLE, to the orders received from her Imperial Majefty,
I fhall endeavour to demonftrate
in a clear and concife manner the deftructive effects of the Small Pox in the natural
way, and the fafety and advantage of
Inoculation, even when performed after the
old manner; and afterwards exhibit the
improvement of the method, being the
fame which is now introduced into this
great empire.

It will not be in my power to execute
this plan with the accuracy I could wifh,
being engaged in an employment that de-
mands much time and attention. But I
will ufe my beft endeavours to defcribe in
the firft place a method of propagating
the practice of Inoculation, fo that it may
not be dangerous to thofe in the neighbourhood, who, either on account of bad
health, age, prejudice, or other reafons,
are unwilling to fubmit to the operation,
and at the fame time render it falutary to
fuch as are proper objects and approve of
it.

It is not to be fuppofed that the method
now practifed in England fo fuccefsfully,
can be received in Ruffia without fome al-
teration. The experiments however which
I have made in England, in order to afcertain the moft commodious manner of
conducting the affair, may be of ufe here;
which I fhall therefore defcribe as clearly
as poffible. * * * * *
* * * * * * *
* * * * * * *
* * * * * * *

In

In the original publifhed in Ruffia, there followed a circumftantial account of the houfe I had built for the accommodation of my patients in England, and the manner of conducting the procefs, &c. there; which, as it would be of no confequence or ufe to infert in this tranflation, I have omitted.

One, and indeed no inconfiderable advantage derived from a plan of this fort is, that by collecting all the patients together in one houfe, the phyfician will be enabled to attend a great number at the fame time in a proper manner, and alfo to pay particular attention to fuch as may more immediately require his affiftance.

And it is of no fmall importance to thofe who have been inoculated, that the neceffary regulations in refpect to regimen, as well as every other circumftance that requires the phyfician's attention, may here be properly obferved.

There

There is likewife another advantage obtained by this method, that, with proper caution, the Small Pox will not be communicated to others in the natural way of infection.

Notwithftanding all thefe conveniencies it will doubtlefs happen here, as it did in my neighbourhood, that many perfons of diftinction will rather prefer the inoculation of their families at their own houfes. In this cafe it is fubmitted to the wifdom of government, whether it would, not be proper to give orders that fuch perfons fhould give public notice of their intention to inoculate, mentioning the time when the operation is to be performed, and alfo of their perfect recovery. By thefe means fuch as have not had the Small Pox, will have it in their power to avoid the infection.

So much with regard to the accommodation of perfons of rank, who may be inoculated under one or the other abovementioned regulations. But the poor cannot enjoy thofe advantages. Humanity how-

however and the intereft of the ftate equally demand, that all poffible attention fhould be beftowed for their affiftance and prefervation.

In order to attain this end, I know of no better or more certain method than that which I followed, on charitable motives only, in my own neighbourhood, by inoculating all the inhabitants of a village who had never had the Small Pox, on the fame day: and, if this be performed in a proper manner, they might be all duly vifited, and proper medicines adminiftered at a moderate expence, and the whole be over in about three weeks: after which, this village would have nothing to apprehend from the Small Pox for fome years. According to this plan, it will be unavoidably neceffary that every child fhould be inoculated for the Small Pox foon after its birth, or that inoculation fhould be performed in every town or village once in five or fix years. This laft method I would rather recommend, and therefore, in order to make this propofal perfectly

in-

intelligible, I shall endeavour to explain it more particularly.

A lift of the names and ages of such inhabitants of every town and village as have not had the Small Pox, is the first neceffary ftep to be taken; and marks should be made againft the names of thofe who on account of their ill ftate of health, or other reafons, are not thought fit fubjects for the operation in the judgment of the inoculator; and fuch perfons should be provided with a feparate place of abode, where they may not be in danger of receiving the infection: the reft fhould be collected together in one place, inoculated at one time, and proper medicines, with directions fpecifying the time and manner in which they are to be taken, fhould be diftributed to each individual. On the fourth day after the inoculation they fhould again be affembled together, the punctures examined, and fuch farther medicines given as the inoculator may think proper. After the feventh the patients fhould be examined daily; for from that time to the eleventh, or perhaps fourteenth, is a period

riod that requires more particular attention. During the whole of this time, and indeed throughout the whole procefs, the fick may continue at their own houfes. And it may be reafonably prefumed, that there will be a fufficient number of fuch as are but flightly indifpofed, who may be able to affift the others, fo as to make the expence and trouble of nurfes unneceffary. But we muft alfo fuppofe, that of the very great number inoculated there will be fome who may have the difeafe feverely, or whofe cafes may require more conftant attendance than they can poffibly have at their own habitations. To provide for fuch extraordinary inftances, therefore, a proper houfe and other conveniencies fhould be previoufly appointed, to which they fhould be removed when thought neceffary.

It will be impoffible to determine precifely how many patients may want fuch attendance, and confequently difficult to provide exactly the neceffary accommodations; but I imagine there will not be
more

more than four or five out of one hundred.

The diet of all fhould confift of vegetables, milk, bread, and the like; and in fome cafes a little mutton-broth may be allowed. The drink fhould be nothing but water, unlefs by the particular direction of the inoculator.

But in order to fecure the obfervance of this regimen more exactly, all falted provifion and every kind of ftrong liquor ought to be removed from the place, and every necefiary precaution taken to prevent the patients from procuring any. In refpect to medicines, the prefcriptions being agreed on by the faculty, a fufficient quantity fhould be prepared, and proper dofes; agreeable to the different age and conftitution, put up feparately, and diftributed by the inoculator among the patients, with directions in what manner they fhould be adminiftered; and their recovery fhould be completed with fome proper purgative.

A li-

A licence or exclufive permiffion ought
to be granted to fuch phyficians or furgeons,
as undertake to inoculate for the Small
Pox; for the mifchief arifing from the
practice of inoculation by the illiterate and
ignorant is beyond conception *. Such
perfons,

---

* To enumerate the inftances that have happened
within my own knowledge to confirm this affertion,
would be almoft endlefs; I fhall only mention a few that
are remarkable.

I was defired to vifit a young woman about ten miles
diftant; I found her dying from the inoculation of a
man, who, upon the credit of having been my coach-
man, had fet up inoculator: he was gone on the pretence
of procuring my affiftance, but in fact had ran away;
this was his thirteenth patient.

Another illiterate perfon in my neighbourhood began
the practice; but a child he had inoculated happening
to have a fit, he was fo frighted as to elope till he was
informed that his patient was out of danger.

I received a letter from a poor man who kept a fchool
about eight miles from Hertford, to inform me, that
not being able to pay a proper perfon, he had ventured to
inoculate his own family himfelf, and begging a vifit on
account of one of his children who he feared was in
danger: I complied with his requeft, and found one
child dying of a confluent pock; but my compaffion
abated, on finding his houfe filled with fome poor neighbours from whom he received a fmall gratuity for their
inoculation, one of which had loft an eye under his

B   care.

perfons, inftead of confining the infection within narrow limits, too often, through want of fkill or honefty, are the means of propagating it, to the great terror of many people, the fatal confequences of which, and the deftructive tokens, remain in many places in England. For befides the dreadful mortality which the difeafe itfelf has occafioned, it has often proved the fource of difcord and contention among neighbours, and difturbed that harmony and friendfhip which had before fubfifted among the inhabitants.

care. This man's refidence was in a fmall town, and from his patients feveral caught the Small Pox, and fome died.

I faw a poor woman dying of a confluent difeafe; her hufband had raifed money for his own inoculation, and having had the difeafe favourably, was affured by a farmer who inoculated him, that he might fafely go home to his family. The wife died, leaving five children, who all had the difeafe and recovered.

At a village not far from Hertford, the fame farmer inoculated as many of the parifh as could raife five fhillings and three-pence, informing the others that the Small Pox was not catching from the inoculated; but the whole neighbourhood became infected, and feveral died.

To

To conclude, I beg this fmall treatife may be confidered only as an imperfect fketch drawn up in hafte; but if it fhould be approved of, and her Imperial Majefty be pleafed to command me to enter into farther particulars, I will employ my utmoft endeavours to render it more perfect, and alfo affift in the execution of any part of what has been therein propofed.

A fhort eftimate of the number of thofe who die of the natural Small Pox, with a view to demonftrate the advantages that may accrue to Ruffia, from the practice of inoculation.

It is needlefs to expatiate upon the havock which the Small Pox makes in moft parts of the known world: probably there is not a country, city, or fmaller community, which has not experienced its devaftations in its turn. The very idea of it is infupportable; but its real effects, in places unapprifed and unacquainted with the proper treatment and remedies againft it, are not lefs general and fatal than the plague itfelf.

B 2   Though

Though this fact is generally allowed, yet many, I think, are ignorant of the immenfe lofs mankind fuftains by this diftemper. It may not be amifs therefore to fhew, from well attefted accounts, the proportion of perfons who die of the natural Small Pox: for which purpofe it will be neceffary to chufe fome country or city where an exact regifter of the births and deaths, as well as an accurate lift of difeafes, is regularly kept.

Dr. Jurin, fecretary to the Royal Society in London, carried this into execution in 1722, foon after Inoculation had been introduced into England, being defirous of fhewing the different effects of the natural and inoculated Small Pox.

I fhall not here infert all that was publifhed by this ingenious author, as the whole may be found in the Philofophical Tranfactions of the Royal Society, under N° 374. The following extract will be fufficient for my prefent purpofe.

The

The Doctor for forty-two years selected from the Bills of Mortality in London, such as died there of the Small Pox and other diftempers. His obfervation may appear perhaps fomewhat extraordinary : neverthelefs he makes it plain, that out of 1000 infants, 386 die under two years of age, which is confiderably more than one third. He then deducts fuch as he fup- pofes die of the difeafes natural to infancy ; and afterwards proceeds to demonftrate, that if the whole bulk of mankind be taken at the age of two years, the eighth part will die of the natural Small Pox ; and that of fuch as have it in the natural way, one in five or fix dies.

With refpect to my own calculations on this fubject, I endeavoured to find out whether the Small Pox proved equally fatal after the time mentioned by the Doctor. With this view, before I left England, I procured the Bills of Morta- lity of the City of London for the laft thirty-four years, excepting two, which could not be found. Of thefe I made a table, which I have added at the end of
this

this treatife. I was furprized to find the number for thefe thirty-two years paft tally fo exactly with the obfervations made by Dr. Jurin.

On examining the table it appears, that within thefe laft thirty-two years 760,098 perfons have died, and of thofe 268,529 have been infants under two years of age, which agrees with Dr. Jurin's calculation, in being rather more than one-third of the whole.

I fuppofe, with Dr. Jurin, that the deaths of thefe were occafioned by different difeafes incidental to infancy, and I deduct them out of the whole number, viz.

$$760,098$$
$$268,529$$

The remainder is 491,569

It appears likewife that in the fame courfe of time there died of the Small Pox 66,515, which confirms Dr. Jurin's account, and indeed exceeds the eighth part. Hence we may fairly conclude, that in general the Small Pox carried off the eighth

part

part of thofe who died in London in the period abovementioned. I procured alfo the beft accounts I poffibly could of the whole number of thofe who had had the difeafe from places where the Small Pox had raged moft, and found, that near one out of five died who had had the difeafe in the natural way. This alfo agrees with Dr. Jurin's obfervations. We fee then that even in London, where the climate is temperate, the difeafe well known, and the treatment of the fick very ably con-ducted, this fingle difeafe deftroyed more than the eighth part of the inhabitants.

But if we turn our eyes towards other dominions, and give credit to the accounts told us, we fhall find the difeafe ftill more fatal, and in fome cities it is almoft as deftructive as the plague.

It is impoffible for me to afcertain with any degree of certainty, the precife num-ber of perfons who die annually of the Small Pox in Ruffia. I am perfuaded however, both from good intelligence as well as my own obfervations, that it is

ex-

exceeding fatal here. Though I cannot confirm this affertion by proofs, yet from fome converfation with the learned I am credibly informed, that of thofe who have the Small Pox in the natural way one-half die, including the rich and poor.

It feems hardly neceffary to fhew, how much the riches and ftrength of ftates depend upon the number of inhabitants. But perhaps there is not any country in which the certainty of this pofition is more indifputable than in Ruffia; for not only the ftrength of the empire, but the riches of every individual alfo, muft be in proportion to the degree of population. If therefore in London, which enjoys the many advantages already recited, more than 2000 perfons die annually of the Small Pox, we may furely fuppofe, that the lofs which Ruffia in its whole extent fuftains by this diftemper in the fame fpace of time, amounts to two millions of fouls. And this havock muft greatly retard the increafe of the human fpecies.

There

There are fome difeafes peculiar to old age, which terminate a life almoft entirely fpent, and totally ufelefs to the community.

Such difeafes, confidered in a political fenfe, are not hurtful to the ftate. But the Small Pox fpreads deftruction chiefly upon the younger part of the fpecies, from whofe labours in their feveral callings the public might otherwife have expected advantages beyond all computation. The difappointment and lofs incurred is of courfe neither to be calculated nor con--ceived.

A difcourfe upon this fubject might be extended to a great length; but it feems unneceffary to enlarge, efpecially when I confider to whofe judgment this effay is with all humility fubmitted.

The public, I am perfuaded, muft be fufficiently convinced from fact and demonftration, that Inoculation is the only means of preventing the mifchiefs arifing from the Small Pox.

C   In

In a former treatife I have laid down a plan for an effectual method of general practice, by which the fpreading of the natural Small Pox will be prevented, and the cure of the inoculated rendered as eafy and fafe as poffible to the patient.

I have therefore nothing more to add but my wifhes, that the empire of Ruffia may meet with the utmoft fuccefs from this difcovery, under the reign of fo il-luftrious and beneficent a Sovereign.

Years.	General List of Deaths.	Deaths from Small Pox.	Under two Years of Age.
1734	26062	2688	10752
35	23538	1594	9672
36	27581	3014	10580
37	27823	2084	10054
38	25825	1590	9600
39			
1740	30811	2725	10765
41	32169	1977	10456
42	27483	1429	9030
43	25200	2029	8621
44	20606	1633	7394
45	21296	1296	7689
46	28157	3236	9503
47	25494	1380	8741
48	23869	1789	7637
49	25516	2625	8504
1750	23727	1229	8204
51	21028	998	7483
52	20485	3538	8239
53	19276	774	7892
54	22696	2359	8115
55	21917	1988	7803
56	20872	1608	7466
57	21313	3296	7095
58	17576	1273	5971
59	19604	2596	6905
1760	19830	2187	6838
61	21063	1525	7699
62	26326	2743	8372
63			
64	23202	2382	7637
65	23230	2498	8073
66	23911	2334	8035
67	22612	2188	7668
	760098	66515	268529

An objection to the practice of Inoculation confidered.

FROM the time that Inoculation was introduced into this country one may date the oppofition to its practice; many learned and ingenious men foon entered the field againft it, and were encountered by others of equal abilities in its defence. The queftions were warmly agitated, and in a fhort time foreigners of great name became authors on both fides. But the ftrength of argument on the part of the defenders of Inoculation, fupported by the good fuccefs of the practice, hath almoft filenced oppofition; and the concurrence of the courts of Peterfburg, Vienna, and France, who have fubmitted to the operation, and by their illuftrious examples encouraged its progrefs in their dominions, will probably clofe the difpute in its favour.

One objection alone feems not to have been fatisfactorily removed, which, although it does not relate to the fafety or health of the patient, is yet of great importance to the community, and well deferves the moft attentive confideration.

You have, fay the objectors, produced accurate and fatisfactory accounts and calculations of the alarming proportion of deaths that happen from the natural Small Pox, and alfo proved, that the lofs fuftained under Inoculation is inconfiderable. But admitting what you have advanced to be true, whence comes it that the fame Bills of Mortality to which you appeal, prove alfo a certain increafe inftead of a diminution of deaths from the Small Pox, and that for fuch a feries of years as to leave no room to difpute the fact? does it not naturally follow, that though almoft the whole number of the inoculated recover, the difeafe muft have been fpread by their means, and a greater proportion having taken the natural difeafe, a confequent greater lofs has been fuftained by the public?

public? If the above is admitted, it will be difficult to exculpate Inoculation from having been hurtful to fociety *.

Se-

* Extract from the Bills of Mortality, and a conti-nuation of the eftimate from page 19.

	Total of Deaths.	Small Pox.	Under 2 Years.			
1768	23639	3028	8229	Total Deaths	178807	
69	21847	1968	8016	Under 2 Years	63056	
70	22434	1986	7994			
71	21780	1660	7617	18821)	115751	(6
72	26053	3992	9112		2825	
73	21656	1039	6850			
74	20884	2479	7742			
75	20514	2669	7496			
	178807	18821	63056	Totals.		

By the above table it will be found, that with refpect to the proportion of infants to the total number of deaths, there is ftill a furprifing agreement with both the former eftimates ; the number of thofe under two years of age remains to be fomewhat more than one-third of the whole.

But if we purfue the fame method as before by fub-ftracting the infants,

$$178807$$
$$63056$$

the number will be 115751

which now amounts to fomewhat more than one in fix; whereas before it was about one in eight.

But

Several attempts have been made to obviate this objection, many of which I have perufed; but confiftent with my intention of brevity, and avoiding all controverfy, I fhall decline entering into particulars, or inferting any quotations from authors. It will be fufficient to fay, that although the arguments advanced have been ingenious, and in fome refpects juft, they do not in my apprehenfion remove the objection that has been mentioned.

Let us fee then whether the practice may not be fairly chargeable with fome blame; and this will appear more evidently, if we take a view of the ufual conduct of families on fuch occafions; which however pertinent to the queftion, feems hitherto to have been avoided, or not attended to, by the feveral writers on the fubject.

But if the eight years are divided, it will appear that the deaths from the Small Pox in the firft four years are 8642; the medium for each of thofe years will be 2166.

For the laft four years the numbers are 10179, the medium for each 2544; an increafe that is truly alarming, and well deferving the attention of the public.— For the *prefent* I fhall forbear any remarks.

In

In London it has been the general custom for thofe who intend to inoculate, to take into account all the circumftances that may be material for the conveniency of their families and friends, and thefe being fettled to their minds, few precautions are thought neceffary refpecting the fecurity of others: what paffes previous to the eruptive fever, does not claim our confideration, fince it is univerfally allowed that no infection can be communicated before that time ; but it is after this period the danger begins, and the difeafe may be fpread by the intercourfe of vifitants, trades people, wafherwomen, fervants, and others, and in a mild ftate of the difeafe, the frequent excurfions of the fick by way of airings, and often in hired carriages of various kinds, contribute greatly towards fpreading the infection. It would perhaps be deemed a defigned omiffion, if the inoculators were not alfo fuppofed to be of the number of thofe that contribute to fpread the difeafe.

When all thefe circumftances are duly confidered, furely it will be allowed, that the

the Small Pox is frequently caught from
the inoculated; and let it be remembered,
that whoever takes the difeafe from an
inoculated patient, has himfelf the natural
Small Pox, with all the circumftances of
danger in refpect to his own life, and of
fpreading the contagion to others.

I know it has been faid, and even pub-
licly declared, that the Small Pox from
Inoculation is fo mild, as fcarcely to be infectious to others; but if this was true,
how comes it that matter, taken from
inoculated patients, conveys the diftemper
with equal certainty, as if it was taken
from the natural Small Pox? is it not
morally certain, that the effluvia partake
of the fame infectious quality? No phyfician of any experience, I am fure, will
ever countenance fuch an opinion. But
left it fhould prevail, and do mifchief
among the ignorant and credulous, I think
it incumbent on me to contradict fo dangerous and unwarrantable an affertion.

In fact, it is certain that the Small Pox
is infectious, in proportion to the number

and

and malignity of the puftules; and fo far there is ufually lefs danger from the artificial difeafe, than from the natural. But let not this prefumption make any ⬛ remit their care, or abate their concern for the community; for I can aſſert from my own knowledge, that * many fatal inftances have happened from the difeafe having been fpread by the inoculated.

Having confidered the fubject as fully as I am able, it fhall be left to the confideration of the public without any comment; only entreating every family that may inoculate, to be extremely careful, and ufe every poffible precaution to prevent fpreading the infection during the illnefs, and to be alfo particularly attentive, that all furniture and cloaths be well aired. The perfons concerned in inoculating fhould, on their parts, take great care that they do not contribute to the mifchief.

If ſtrict attention is paid to thefe particulars, it may be reafonably hoped, that

* Vide note page 9.

the

the only remaining objection to the practice of Inoculation in London among perſons of condition, may be much weakened, if not entirely removed.

On

On general and partial Inoculations in the country.

THE preceding tranflated treatifes having been calculated for Ruffia, which in many circumftances differs from England, and in particular that the will of the Sovereign there is moft implicitly obeyed, cannot be expected to contain all that may be neceffary to be confidered, and attended to in this country.

Neverthelefs, the general principle of the regulation, fo far as it relates to public Inoculation in towns and villages, may be attended to, and of fuch places I mean to treat firft, and of London and other populous places afterwards, for reafons that will be fufficiently evident in the fequel.

In order to be fully acquainted with the fubject, it feems neceffary to take into confideration, the mode of conducting this affair in the country, which I do not remember

member to have ever feen circumftantially publifhed; thofe who have wrote on the fubject, having for the moft part contented themfelves with reprefentations of their fuccefs only.

In the county of Hertford, there have been two methods of public or general Inoculation, one to inoculate, at a low price, as many of the inhabitants of any fmall town or village, as could be perfuaded to fubmit to it, and at the fame time were able to pay, refufing all thofe who had it not in their power to procure the money demanded.

The other method has been, where the inhabitants of a town, or diftrict, of all denominations, have agreed to be inoculated at the fame time, the parifh officers, or fome neighbouring charitably difpofed perfons, having firft promifed to defray the expence, and provide fubfiftance for fuch of the poor, as were unable to pay for themfelves.

The

The partial method firſt mentioned has been attended by much miſchief, and ſufficiently refuted the abſurd opinion endeavoured to be propagated by intereſted perſons, that inoculated perſons do not communicate infection; innumerable are the inſtances which have happened of the diſeaſe being caught from the inoculated, and too evident to be denied; and ſo many of theſe have died, that an opinion not leſs abſurd than the former prevails in Hertfordſhire, that thoſe who take the Small Pox from the inoculated rarely recover.

The method of inoculating every one in the ſame neighbourhood together has ſucceeded ſo happily, that it ſeems only neceſſary to determine what is the moſt reaſonable and frugal way of conducting the buſineſs; and if joined to this conſideration proper attention is paid to airing and cleanſing the patients, their cloaths and habitations, as much as poſſible, from the power of infection, all the benefit that can be derived from general Inoculation will be effected, many valuable lives will be preſerved to the community, and the inhabitants

habitants made happy, on being releafed from the apprehenfions of a vifit from this cruel difeafe.

As I can from confiderable experience fpeak with fome confidence on this fubject, I fhall proceed to relate the obfervations that have occurred to me. Affifted by my learned friend Dr. Ingenhouz and my two fons, I inoculated, at different times, the neighbouring parifhes of Eaft Berkhamfted, Hertingfordbury, Bayford, and the liberty of Brickenden; in each of thefe places the whole number of poor were inoculated, with the exception of thofe who were ob-jectionable. I do not at prefent remember the exact number, I believe they might be more than 600; but know that they fuc-ceeded happily, though there were feveral very old perfons, and women in different periods of geftation; and this mode of practice, as I have been informed, has been alfo ufed fuccefsfully by many others in different parts of England.

So far as has come to my knowledge, general Inoculations have hitherto been
confined

confined to fmall towns and villages; yet as the further extenfion is very much to be wifhed, it may not be improper to relate fome particulars of what paffed in Hertford, which is doubtlefs the largeft, and moft populous town, that has fubmitted to the experiment, of inoculating at the fame time the whole number of its inhabitants.

In a former publication, I gave an account of the occafion and fuccefs of a general Inoculation at this place; from that time the town was releafed from any apprehenfions of the difeafe, until the year 1770, when it appeared again, and two or three having died, a few perfons were inoculated, and excited an alarm. On this occafion, the poor in my neighbourhood flocked in numbers, befeeching me to extend to them the fame charitable affiftance, they had formerly experienced; having then my two fons with me to affift, I complied without hefitation.

Nothing fhews the increafe and ftate of population fo clearly, as an experiment of this kind; we had then upwards of two hundred

hundred and fifty patients, fome of whom were new inhabitants, but the reft confifted for the moft part of very young children. Neceffity has often produced ufeful difcoveries; the Inoculation was begun on Midfummer-day, and though the weather proved very hot, I obferved no inconvenience from it; they had the free ufe of air, and feemed as much benefited by it as at any other feafon of the year; and every one recovered.

In the year 1774 the difeafe appeared a third time; the fame requeft was renewed, and with the fame affiftance afforded, the whole town was inoculated once more, and now the number amounted only to about one hundred and twenty; from that time we have heard nothing of Small Pox, and I verily believe, that within thefe ten years not fix perfons have died in Hertford of this difeafe; whereas before the practice was fo generally adopted, the Small Pox has frequently been epidemic and deftroyed a great number of the inhabitants, befides injuring the market and trade of the town for a confiderable time.

E   The

The inferences one may fairly draw from thefe premifes are, that in fmall towns or villages, if fome are inoculated and others excluded, unlefs more precautions are ufed than may reafonably be apprehended, the confequence will be, that the difeafe will fpread through the vicinage, and be fatal to many.

On the contrary, if by general confent a public Inoculation is agreed on, and the poor are fupplied with neceffaries, the happieft confequences may be reafonably expected; and further, the good effect of repeated general Inoculations in the town of Hertford demonftrate, that large towns may. with great advantage avail themfelves of the fame means, and, by occafionally repeating the practice, be fecured from the ravages of this juftly dreaded difeafe,

On general and partial Inoculations
in London, or other large and populous places.

IT fhould be remarked, that what has hitherto been faid relates to the conduct of
this practice in villages and fmall towns,
who are capable of uniting in a general
plan for their common benefit. What I
next propofe to confider is, how far a
practicable method can be adopted for general Inoculation in London, or in other
large and populous places, where it is impoffible to obtain the confent of all the
inhabitants to be inoculated at one and
the fame time.

To be the more clearly underftood, I
defire the diftinction in the former part of
general and partial Inoculations may be remembered; and that by the firft I mean,
where the whole number of inhabitants of
any town or place are inoculated at the
fame time, with the exception only of

E 2   fuch

such as are not in a proper state of health, and those who may not chuse to submit to that mode of receiving the disease. By the second, where a part only of the inhabitants are inoculated, and the remainder left to take their chance of catching the disease from their inoculated neighbours.

The possibility of performing a general Inoculation on all the inhabitants of this city and suburbs at one time, will scarce bear a moment's consideration, so many and so insuperable are the difficulties which would occur in a free country. I shall therefore decline entering upon the subject; and quitting all thoughts of a general practice, shall consider how far the inoculation of such poor persons as may make application for this purpose, can be complied with in London, consistent with the safety of themselves and others.

It may reasonably be presumed, that the greater number of these will be persons in narrow circumstances, or in a state of poverty, having nothing beforehand to support an illness, and yet the whole family who

who have not had the difeafe are to be inoculated. Whoever has vifited the abodes of the poor in and about London, muft allow the fcene to be truly miferable; their habitations in clofe alleys, courts, and lanes, generally cold, dirty, and in great want of neceffaries, even of bedding itfelf, a requifite of the greateft ufe in time of ficknefs; there are frequently feveral families under one roof; the men, if induftrious, employed in daily labour, the women in wafhing and affifting in different families, or waiting at markets to carry little burdens as porters, and other unavoidable employments abroad. None of thefe can remit their occupations to attend the fick, without expofing their families to the diftrefs which the want of the little money their induftry earned would infallibly occafion; how or in what manner are patients to be nurfed and fupplied with food and neceffaries during the illnefs, or who is to be relied on, that the medicines and diet enjoined by the perfon who attends, fhall be regularly complied with?

Can

Can any one be so inconsiderate as to bring disease into a family before healthy, without having first a reasonable expectation, that what their situation may require will certainly be provided? no one acquainted with the general temper of parish officers, will much depend on their assistance; on the contrary, they will most probably oppose the plan to the utmost of their endeavours, from an apprehension that the disease will be spread by these means, and occasion a consequent increase of expence to the parish.

But admitting these objections could be removed, one very important point, that more immediately respects the security of the patients and the public, should be attended to.

One great cause of the success that attends the present practice, is supposed to be the exposure of patients to fresh air; and the more alarming the symptoms, the greater is the necessity of administering this salutary relief. The poor who are inoculated in their own confined dwellings,

4   with

with perhaps many in family, will affuredly require this reviving ventilation. They have no gardens, areas, or the convenience of carriages; are they to be carried or led about the ftreets when ill, to the terror and danger of the neighbourhood?

Having fuggefted a few of the difficulties that muft enfue to the patients, it will not be improper to confider, how far the community will be likely to be affected by the practice.

To conduct the bufinefs of the Inoculation, fome place or places centrically fituated muft be provided, at which the patients fhould affemble in order to be inoculated, and to which the feveral families of the fick muft have recourfe for the neceffary medicines and directions during the diftemper. To find one or more fuch places in the whole city, where the neighbourhood would fuffer an office of this kind to be eftablifhed, at which a great number of the poor muft be affembled at noon-day, to receive an infectious and dangerous difeafe, is hardly poffible to conceive; and if

we

we confider that thefe perfons muft inter-
mix with others, who are attending to procure the neceffary medicines for their dif-
eafed families, and who have been obliged
to make their way on foot through the
public ftreets, from every quarter of the
metropolis, in their infected apparel, the
public danger becomes great and inevi-
table.

But fhould the poor who are proper to
undergo the operation be inoculated, and
means for their fubfiftence be provided,
queftions will arife refpecting the fate of
their neighbours, fome of whom will be
precluded from the fame advantage, by
being affected with other difeafes, and others,
who have ftrong prejudices againft it, will
be totally averfe to the practice. Is it rea-
fonable to bring the Small Pox to the doors
of perfons thus circumftanced, againft their
confent? one fhudders at the thought of
fuch an infult to humanity! But it is not
only the immediate neighbours that would
be endangered; to be well informed how
far the mifchief might be extended, one
muft take into account the fituation and
conduct

conduct of the patients, and it may fafely be afferted from experience, that the following would be found to be a true reprefentation.

The inoculated may be divided into two clafles. One in whom the diftemper is fo mild as to admit the parties to go abroad; the other, where the number of puftules is fo confiderable as to confine the patients at home; by far the greater number will be of the firft fort; and whatever orders may be given to the contrary, it will be impoffible to reftrain them from taking undue liberties; the children who are of an age for it will be found in the ftreets with their former playfellows, and the men and women who are able, will be endeavouring to get into their former employments to earn a little money, without regarding the injury they may occafion to others. The few who may be confined with a lefs favourable difeafe, will infect the houfe and their family, and the infection will be fpread from the goffiping difpofition of the poor, who are generally troublefome vifitants, to their fick neighbours, and after

F   all

all is over, the firft fallying forth in their
infected cloaths is certain to add to the
mifchief.

It is unneceffary to dwell any longer on
the confequences of fuch a conduct to the
refidents in fuch alleys; but there are
others who claim our regard.

Country people who are obliged to come
to town to tranfact their bufinefs, and
others who bring their families to vifit re-
lations, or to entertain them with the
pleafures of the town, are generally under
dreadful apprehenfions of the Small Pox;
how would their fears and danger be increafed, if the poor were continually under
inoculation ?

Another thoughtlefs, but moft ufeful
race of men, are well entitled to our beft
endeavours for the prefervation of their
healths and lives: I mean, failors and fea-
faring men, of our own and other coun-
tries; it is well known that our fhores,
on both fides of the river, are continually
crouded

crouded with thefe, during their ftay in this country.

Many of them have not had the Small Pox, and their mode of living is the reverfe of due preparation; if Inoculation fhould be practifed in the houfes of the poor, it cannot be doubted that many of thefe would catch this diftemper?

Is it poffible to reflect without horror on the fituation of fuch of thofe unhappy fellows, who fhould fall ill of the Small Pox in the miferable lodgings they ufually inhabit, perhaps without a friend to take the leaft care of them? or of the ftill more calamitous ftate of others, who being infected on fhore fhould fall fick at fea, where neither medicine nor proper attendance can be had, and carry likewife with them in their unwafhed cloaths, the fatal diftemper into diftant climates?

I have been informed, that a child who had received the infection was taken on board an Eaft Indiaman many years ago. The difeafe was violent; the linen, &c.

were

were put into a box, and carried to the
Cape of Good Hope: it was fent on fhore;
the Small Pox immediately broke out in
the place, and carried off vaft numbers of
the inhabitants.

In the foregoing pages, fome of the objections to partial Inoculations of the poor
in this city have been ftated; but the pof-
fibility of extending the practice to any
good purpofe, even if thofe objections were
removed, has not been taken notice of:
to elucidate this point, which is certainly
a material one, the following remarks are
fubmitted to confideration.

The number of thofe who died of the
Small Pox in each of the laft four years,
on an average is 2544. To fuppofe that
one dies out of every fix who have the natural diftemper, will be allowed a moderate
eftimate: it follows then, that the number
of thofe who have paffed through the difeafe in each of the laft four years will be
15,264. It will be impoffible to determine
how many may remain uninfected; but if
we fuppofe that every year one out of eight

6   who

who have not had the difeafe is feized with it, the remaining number who have not had the Small Pox will be 122,112; and it muft be taken into account, that the annual recruits by births will probably be about 20,000, befides others that are continually arriving out of the country to feek employment.

To form a fcheme, however beneficial to a few, that would probably fpread the difeafe, and involve fo great a number of others in a danger that they would otherwife be much lefs expofed to, is an object of great moment; and moft certainly the Legiflature ought firft to be confulted.

Great liberty may be taken in our free ftate; but we ought not to endanger the public fafety, becaufe no legal provifion is made againft it.

Of

Of an Hofpital for Inoculation.

IF the objections that have been noticed fhould be deemed of fufficient force to fet afide all thoughts of partial Inoculations of the poor in London, what is to be done will next become the queftion? It would be cruel and unreafonable to refufe the benefit of this difcovery to the neceffi-tous, who on that very account are moft intitled to our affiftance; yet how to pro-vide for them, confiflent with the fafety of their neighbours, feems difficult, though I hope not impracticable.

A defire to fee fome expedient for this purpofe fucceed, induces me to fubmit to the confideration of the public, a propofal that is in my apprehenfion liable to few ob-jections, and would beft anfwer the pur-pofe.

It is to eftablifh an Hofpital for the pur-pofe of Inoculation only.

I am,

I am aware that Hofpitals have been ftigmatized as unhealthy, from the idea that a number of fick perfons confined together corrupt the air, and generate contagious putrid difeafes. This charge has, I think, been inconfideratcly made, fo far as relates to Hofpitals in and near this metropolis; but as it is no part of my undertaking to difpute the point, I fhall confine myfelf to what concerns an Hofpital for Inoculation, which, if every circumftance is duly attended to, will be as little unhealthy as any houfe in the kingdom.

Let us for a moment drop the offenfive name of Hofpital, and fuppofe a large houfe is provided in a healthy fituation, with convenient and airy apartments for the reception of any given number of perfons capable of being commodioufly contained in it; that to be in a good ftate of health would be the neceffary qualification on the admiffion of every perfon, and about three weeks the time of the refidence; and that the difeafe they are to undergo is ufually fo mild, as to permit moft of the patients to be abroad in the open air almoft

every

every day, and of a nature not to communicate any putrid injury to others, except its own fpecific poifon. If to thefe circumftances we add, that the patients will in general be children and young perfons, that their cloaths and apartments will be clean, and their food wholefome and fuch as is proper for their condition, furely one may boldly affert, that a family thus circumftanced will have the faireft profpect of enjoying good health.

Having endeavoured to remove the prejudice that is apt to accompany the idea of an Hofpital fo far as relates to health, I fhall proceed to enumerate the advantages that will moft probably be obtained by an inftitution of this kind; fome of thefe have been already mentioned in the tranflation, and I fhall take the liberty of introducing them again in this place, with little variation, as they relate to the fubject.

" One, and indeed no inconfiderable advantage to be derived from a plan of this fort will be, that all the patients being collected together in one houfe, the phyfician

fician will be enabled to attend a great number at the fame time in a proper manner, and can be particularly attentive to fuch as may more immediately require his affiftance.

" And it is of no fmall importance to thofe who are inoculated, that the neceffary regulations in refpect to regimen, as well as every other circumftance that requires the phyfician's attention, will be there properly obferved, and the neceffary medicines always at hand, with an able perfon to direct the manner ~~that~~ they ought to be adminiftered.

" There is likewife another advantage obtained by this method, that with proper caution the Small Pox will not be communicated to others in the natural way of infection.

It is alfo an encouraging circumftance, that an eftablifhment of this fort will be attended with lefs expence, in feveral particulars, than any other Hofpital.

G " One

One phyfician will be able to fuper-
intend the procefs of Inoculation in a very
great number of patients, provided he is
affifted by a refident apothecary to receive
his inftruction, and to be at hand to affift
on extraordinary emergencies.

Few drugs or medicines will be
wanted; the expence therefore on the articles will be very trifling.

Few attendants on the fick will be neceffary, and not fo much as one under the
character of a nurfe; for there will always
be a fufficient number of patients in fo
good a ftate of health, as to be able to attend on thofe who may require affiftance;
and it fhould be one condition of their ad-
mittance, that they fhould be willing to
affift others when able, as they would wifh
to be attended themfelves when they ftand
in need of it; and if this injunction is
complied with, it may be expected that
there will be a fufficient number in a ftate
of health to perform this office for one
another. The doing the heavy and dirty
part of the work, the care of the children,
the

the attendance of thofe who may have the difeafe more feverely, and the bufinefs of the kitchen, will doubtlefs require a proper number of healthy maid-fervants.

In refpect to diet, as it will be chiefly of the vegetable and leaft expenfive kinds of food, this will be a very moderate article in the œconomy of fuch an eftablifhment."

On

On the Hospitals at Pancras.

THE Hospitals for Small Pox in the natural way and Inoculation were instituted in 1746, and have been supported by voluntary subscription.

These Hospitals consist of two houses at a sufficient distance from each other, and in airy situations.

That for preparing the patients for inoculation at Pancras contains 100 beds; and that for receiving them when the disease appears, and for admitting those who are seized with the Small Pox in the natural way, in Cold Bath Fields, 130 beds.

All who are destitute of friends or money and are attacked with this disease, or are desirous of being inoculated, if seven years old or upwards, are proper objects of this charity.

Patients

Patients in the natural way are received every day, if there is room for them; and to prevent the danger and expence of a difappointment, enquiry fhould be firft made. Patients for Inoculation are alfo received every day at Pancras before nine in the morning.

Strangers are forbid to vifit the patients.

Cloaths are provided for the patients, while their own cloaths are freed from infection before their difcharge.

As the firft outline of every attempt towards a new inftitution has for the moft part been imperfect, it is not to be wondered at if the plan and regulations of thefe Hofpitals fhould admit of improvements; and the following remarks will perhaps point out fome regulations that deferve attention.

It is now near thirty years fince the firft eftablifhment of this charity; at which time it was the received opinion that a ftrict regimen ought to be obferved, and a

courfe

courfe of medicine complied with, by way
of preparing the moft healthy previous to
their Inoculation. It was alfo believed,
that there was fome rifque of taking the
natural infection injurioufly at the time of
being inoculated, and danger of accumulation by refiding with others who had the
difeafe; and the inoculators of that time
who made ufe of infected thread and lint,
fometimes failed infecting on the firft trial,
and in fuch cafe the patient would probably
catch the natural diftemper by cohabiting
with the fick.

Thefe opinions, it is prefumed, joined
with the defign of admitting patients in
the natural Small Pox, determined the firft
Governors to have two Hofpitals; one, to
contain all fuch who were actually under-
going the difeafe in either way, and in a
ftate to infect others: the other to be ap-
propriated to fuch only who were under
preparation, or having been inoculated had
as yet no appearance of the ufual eruptive
fymptoms, and were not in a condition to
infect one another. But thefe opinions
have not been verified by experience; on
the

the contrary, it has turned out that the precautions were not neceffary. Experience affures us, that a perfon in good health may be fafely inoculated without any preparation, and that all the regulations in refpect to diet and the neceffary courfe of medicine, may be fufficiently complied with in the week that intervenes between the operation and the commencement of the difeafe. With refpect to a double infection, that is, by Inoculation and in the ufual courfe of communication, or an accumulation of the diftemper afterwards by living with thofe who are actually labouring under it, no ill confequence need be feared; for I am perfectly fatisfied, that after Inoculation is effectually performed, no injury can be fuftained by living with others in the moft infectious ftate. And even if the firft Inoculation fhould fail infecting (which if proper care is taken will fcarce ever happen) the failure may be difcovered on the third or fourth day, and the patient may be inoculated again; and even then, fhould there be a moral certainty that the natural infection has been taken, it will be in time to prevent any ill effects;

effects; the inoculated difeafe will as it were fupercede and annihilate the former infection, and the patient have the Small Pox from Inoculation only.

I am aware that fome apology is neceffary on publifhing opinions that may be deemed improbable in fo laconic a manner; this is no place to purfue the fubject; but I mean foon to fupport thefe affertions by relating certain facts on which they are founded. It is probable, that from a deliberate confideration of thefe circumftances, fome confiderable improvements may be made in the regulations of the Hofpital.

A principal one fhould be, to quit the practice of bringing the inoculated patients to refide with thofe who have the natural difeafe; a circumftance that could not have been confented to but from the former miftaken opinions which have been noticed. A confiderable advantage will alfo be gained to the œconomy of the Hofpital, on account of the time of the patients refidence being fhortened; by which means a greater

4   number

number may be inoculated at the fame expence.

I hope to ftand excufed from having
made thefe remarks here, as in the fequel
I mean to propofe an enlargement of the
Hofpital at Pancras.

. Having taken notice of the moft material articles that have occurred relative to
this fubject, I fhall venture, though with
much diffidence, to fubmit fome outlines
of an Hofpital for Inoculation to the public, premifing, that in refpect to fituation,
the environs of London do not feem to
afford a better fpot than that on which the
inoculating Hofpital at Pancras is built,
which, with the ground adjoining to it
being four acres, is fufficient for the accommodation of any number of patients
for the benefit of the air; in fhort, every
local advantage would be there enjoyed in
great perfection : the prefent building is
not however capacious enough for fuch a
purpofe, but it may be enlarged, and the
whole extent of ground ought to be walled

H   in,

in, to prevent all intercourse with others, or giving any offence to the public; and I have not the least doubt of the acquiescence and assistance of the present governors, to any scheme for the extension of this noble and useful charity, as they have, with a most distinguished application and disinterestedness, employed their best endeavours to promote the interest of the present establishment.

But previous to every other step, an application to Parliament for encouragement, and proper powers to carry this design into execution, seems necessary; for it will not be sufficient to open an Hospital for Inoculation, without offering something as an inducement to invite those who are proper objects to accept of the benefits intended. Amongst the lower classes of people in the metropolis, as well as in many other places, the voice of the generality is against Inoculation; prejudices are not easily removed; nor is it to be expected that the many will attend to the advantages that will result to their children, unless unlefs fome prefent benefits were to be connected with them *.

If parifh officers were obliged by Act of Parliament to apply to the Hofpital for the admiffion of every man or woman who fhould either on their own account, or on behalf of their children, exprefs a defire of being inoculated, and on their being taken in to fupply each with two new fhirts or fhifts, and fign an obligation to provide decent new cloathing for every one on their receiving notice of their recovery

---

* While the Emprefs was under Inoculation at Sarfco-ceio, fome of the poor of the adjoining village were alfo, on the encouragement fhe had given, inoculated.

I remember the Emprefs faid to me, with that vivacity and liberality of fentiment for which fhe is remarkably diftinguifhed, " If I was to order the poor of this neighbourhood to be inoculated, it would be complied with, and be beneficial to them; but I love to ufe perfuafive means, rather than authority; on this account I have advanced a rouble (about four fhillings) to each that would confent, and feveral have accepted it and recovered; but I find they now talk of raifing the price to two roubles, which I muft confent to as a further encouragement, for I wifh the practice may be advanced by the mildeft methods."

and

and time of difmiffion, and alfo to give a
fmall gratuity (fuppofe half a crown) to
every perfon of the age of   and
to the parents of every child, on producing
a certificate of their having behaved de-
cently, and complied with the rules of the
houfe, figned by the phyfician, it would
probably be a fufficient inducement, and
at the fame time the frefh cloathing would
effectually prevent the fpreading the difeafe
to others.   And this could not be reafonably deemed a hardfhip, fince fome of the
moft refpectable old Hofpitals exact as
much on admiffion of parifh patients *.

It is fcarcely to be doubted but that
Parliament would cheerfully embrace a
plan of this nature, which has for its object the prefervation of the lives of the
poor, and carrying them and their children

---

* At St. Thomas's Hofpital, every patient on admiffion pays 2s. 6d. if clean, or 10s. 6d. if venereal;
and the overfeer or churchwarden of the parifh figns an
obligation that he will find clean body linen every week,
and pay four pence a day fo long as he continues in the
Hofpital, and receive him when difcharged, or take
away the body, or pay the burial fees to the fteward of
the Hofpital, in cafe of death.

safely through this terrible difeafe, without endangering their neighbourhoods.

Parifhes would likewife find their account in it: by a known moderate charge they would be releafed from the contingent great expence of maintaining many fick families, occafionally afflicted with the Small Pox in the natural way; oftentimes to the great injury of trade and manufactures: and this by a trifling advance to be beftowed but once during the life of an individual, who would be maintained about three weeks without any further expence, and return home to wear the cloaths they had beftowed on him.

Thus much I have thought neceffary to ftate, from a moral certainty that fome provifion of this fort fhould be made; to proceed, would be entering into minute matters that would more properly belong to the governors, who will be beft able to make fuch regulations as may be for the general benefit of the charity.

So

So much has already been said on general Inoculations in the country, that it seems unneceffary to enter on the fubject again in this place. But fuch is the obftinacy of fome parifhes, and the parfimony of others, that it is impoffible for the poor who are defirous of being inoculated, to perfuade them to advance the fmall fum that would be neceffary to defray the expence; and they are therefore obliged to wait the event of the natural difeafe, while the principal inhabitants are fecuring their own families by Inoculation.

Another unjuftifiable piece of frugality that deferves attention and to be remedied is, that in many places where the whole number of poor have been inoculated at the expence of the parifh, illiterate fellows, totally unacquainted with difeafes or remedies, have been employed on account of cheapnefs only; when at the fame time the families of the wealthy have been under the care of medical gentlemen of good reputation. To infert all the inftances that might be produced of parochial meannefs would be tedious; I fhall
mention

mention the following only, which may be relied on as an indisputable truth. The inhabitants of a certain parish had a meeting to agree on inoculating all the poor; some medical gentlemen in the neighbourhood offered to undertake the business at a very low price; but as cheapness was the only object of consideration, the parish was about to agree with a black-smith at eighteen pence a head, when one of the most frugal started this objection: It is very probable that under this man's care we may have some die, and the expence of their burial may cost the parish so much, that it might be as well to agree with a better man. This objection was thus removed by the smith :—" Come, I'll tell " you what I'll do with you.—Give me half " a crown a head, and them that die I will " carry to the church-yard without putting " the parish to any further expence."

Thus to trifle with the lives of their indigent fellow creatures, must be an indelible reproach to any people. I know it will be said, that many instances can be produced, where whole parishes of poor have

have been inoculated, and have fucceeded very well, under the care of perfons who were totally unacquainted with medicine.

I will not here difpute the truth of this affertion; and indeed, if it was not an eafy matter to procure more able help, it might be better to continue the practice in that way than to neglect inoculating entirely; but this is not the cafe. Gentlemen of the profeffion of good abilities will go very low in their price; and when it is confidered that the fum is to be paid but once in the life of each perfon, furely parifhes ought to be compelled to employ one who has had a medical education, and others fhould be reftrained to their own proper bufinefs.

But it happens not unfrequently that irregular and dangerous fymptoms appear, and at other times a different difeafe attacks the patient at the fame time, with fome unufual complaints while under Inoculation; thefe fituations would certainly require the affiftance of a perfon who could judge well of the fymptoms, and diftinguifh guiſh the diſeaſes properly, and know how to treat them, which a man unacquainted with the principles or the practice of phyſic could not pretend to, and conſequently the patient would be expoſed to great danger. Should an Act of Parliament be procured, it would be neceſſary to provide for the following circumſtances.

That every pariſh (with the exception of ſuch large places as ſhould be thought too populous to be included) ſhould be enjoined to offer Inoculation to all their poor who ſhould be willing to admit of it *; that the patients and their families ſhould be maintained during their illneſs; that the perſon employed to inoculate ſhould have had ſome education in medicine as phyſician, ſurgeon, or apothecary; and that once in five years the ſame offer ſhould be renewed, leaving the time of year and other circumſtances to the option of the pariſh.

* Vide Page 3, &c;

I   Iƒ

If thefe obligatory claufes were obtained,
general Inoculations in the country might
be carried on at a very moderate expence.

C O N-

CONCLUSION.

ON a review of what has been advanced it will appear, that the practice of Inoculation has been upon the whole rather hurtful than advantageous to the city of London, and that the mortality from Small Pox has lately increased to an alarming degree: that it may be presumed this loss has not been sustained by the wealthy, who have availed themselves of their easy circumstances, and by timely Inoculation have secured their families; but that the loss has fallen principally among those who are not the least useful members of the community, viz. on young persons, the offspring of inferior trades-people, and the labouring poor.

It has been shewn, that to encourage partial Inoculations among such of the poor as might be willing to accept the offer, and should be found in a proper state of health, would be to increase the evil, by

spreading

spreading the disease in a destructive manner among their neighbours, and be on
other accounts dangerous and intolerable.
An hospital for the purpose of Inoculation *only* has been rescued from the unjust
charge of being unhealthy, and has been
proved to enjoy superior advantages in that
respect, and many others; and that a well-
regulated plan of this kind would effectually answer the purposes of abating the
mortality, and securing the community
from being infected by the patients.

An application therefore to the Legisla-
ture for approbation and assistance seems
highly expedient; and it is not to be
doubted but the generous and humane
would readily be induced to raise by subscription a fund sufficient to carry these
good designs into execution; so that as we
are the first European nation who received
and encouraged Inoculation, we may also
have the honour of being the first who
have generously diffused the benefit of it to
the community at large, and transmitted
it to posterity.

We

We have thus far only taken into confideration what refpects the two extremes of fociety, the opulent and indigent; but there ftill remains a numerous and refpectable part of the community unnoticed, I mean, perfons who are in but moderate circumftances, yet above accepting the charity of an hofpital.

Perfons thus circumftanced feem to have a claim upon the humanity of fuch practitioners as are eminent in their profeffion; who, from that motive, we doubt not, will chearfully give their attendance on fuch terms as families can afford. By this well-timed generofity, the minds of the middle rank of people will be made eafy, and it will be a great inducement for them alfo to inoculate their families.

To conclude, I have ufed my beft endeavours to reprefent the whole that has been treated of in its true light, and recommended the methods that have feemed to me to anfwer the purpofes moft effectually. It may probably happen, that zeal in the caufe may have carried me too far,

4

or that through inadvertency fome errors may have been made. If they are pointed out, I will acknowledge them with thanks to the informer, having nothing more in view than the good of the public, and that the practice recommended may be fo conducted as to afford its oppofers as few objections, on any folid ground, as pof-fible.

It is fo truly the caufe of humanity, and fo certain of anfwering the purpofe, that I moft earneftly recommend a liberal fupport to all charitably difpofed perfons, and more efpecially to fuch in affluent circumftances, who may have experienced the happy effects of Inoculation in their own families, concluding with the words conftantly ufed by a beggar in Turky,

WHAT THOU DOEST, THOU DOEST TO THYSELF.

FINIS.